VEGETARIAN JOURNAL

DATE: ____________________

TIME: ____________________

DATE: ____________________

TIME: ____________________

DATE: ____________________

TIME: ____________________

DATE: ____________

TIME: ____________

DATE: ____________________

TIME: ____________________

DATE: ____________________

TIME: ____________________

DATE: ____________________

TIME: ____________________

DATE: ____________________

TIME: ____________________

DATE: ____________________

TIME: ____________________

DATE: ____________________

TIME: ____________________

DATE: ______________________

TIME: ______________________

DATE: ____________________

TIME: ____________________

DATE: ____________________

TIME: ____________________

DATE: ____________________

TIME: ____________________

DATE: ____________________

TIME: ____________________

DATE: ____________________

TIME: ____________________

DATE: ____________________

TIME: ____________________

DATE: ____________________

TIME: ____________________

DATE: __________________

TIME: __________________

DATE: ______________

TIME: ______________

DATE: ____________________

TIME: ____________________

DATE: ____________________

TIME: ____________________

DATE: ____________________

TIME: ____________________

DATE: ______________________

TIME: ______________________

DATE: ____________________

TIME: ____________________

DATE: ____________________

TIME: ____________________

DATE: ____________________

TIME: ____________________

DATE: ____________________

TIME: ____________________

DATE: ___________________

TIME: ___________________

DATE: ________________

TIME: ________________

DATE: ______________________

TIME: ______________________

DATE: ____________________

TIME: ____________________

DATE: ____________________

TIME: ____________________

DATE: ____________________

TIME: ____________________

DATE: ____________________

TIME: ____________________

DATE: ____________________

TIME: ____________________

DATE: ____________________

TIME: ____________________

DATE: ____________________

TIME: ____________________

DATE: ____________________

TIME: ____________________

DATE: ____________________

TIME: ____________________

DATE: ____________________

TIME: ____________________

DATE: ____________________

TIME: ____________________

DATE: ____________________

TIME: ____________________

DATE: ____________________

TIME: ____________________

DATE: ____________________

TIME: ____________________

DATE: ____________________

TIME: ____________________

DATE: ____________________

TIME: ____________________

DATE: ____________________

TIME: ____________________

CPSIA information can be obtained
at www.ICGtesting.com
Printed in the USA
LVHW061024210723
752765LV00012B/433